Uncovering Fibromyalgia

By

Lynne D M Noble

Copyright 2019 Lynne D M Noble

This book shall not, by way of trade or otherwise, be lent, re-sold, hired out, or otherwise circulated without the prior consent of the copyright holder or the publisher in any form of binding or cover than that in which it is published and without a similar condition including this condition being imposed on the subsequent purchaser.

The use of its contents in another media is also subject to the same conditions.

Independently published 2019

About the Author

Lynne Noble was born in 1953 in Huddersfield, West Yorkshire. From a very early age, Lynne showed an interest in nutrition and genetics avidly reading any books that she could get her hands on at the time.

Initially, Lynne studied orthopaedics but events led her to work with the elderly mentally infirm. Here, her interest in neurodegenerative disorders and pain syndromes developed.

Lynne undertook rigorous programmes of study, completing her Cert Ed., (FE) BSc (Hons) and Adv. Dip Education simultaneously before moving onto her M.Ed.

From there she took further demanding programmes in Human Nutrition, Pharmacology, Neuroscience, Genetics and Immunology. During this time, she was given many prestigious awards for her academic work. It was noted then that Lynne was not afraid of tackling difficult subjects.

She began her law degree but ill health prevented her from pursuing this. However, in this time, she moved from being a foster parent to adoptive parent.

She has been instrumental in setting up projects in the community for disadvantaged groups.

She is a member of the Guild of Health Writers.

Now retired, she lives in a picturesque village in West Yorkshire with her husband. She enjoys gardening, watching her husband bowling and researching.

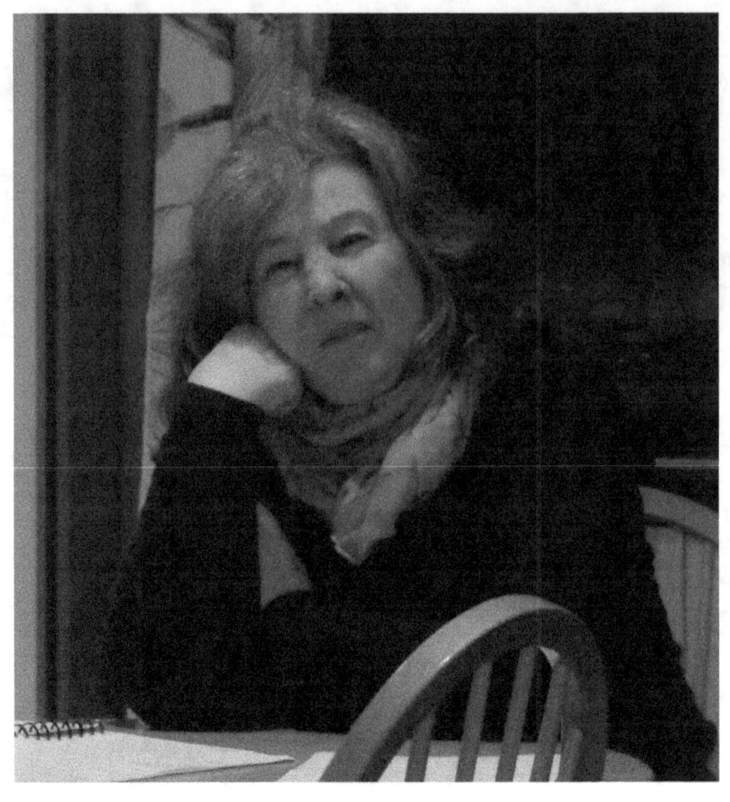

Author Lynne Noble at home

https://quintessentiallylynne.weebly.com/nutritional-medicine.html

Contents

Preface

Fibromyalgia syndrome must be one of the most misunderstood conditions. It was recognised in 1981 and the first set of guidelines for its diagnosis appeared in 1988, more or less at the same time that chronic fatigue syndrome was recognised.

It was viewed with suspicion by many in governmental departments who saw these new kids on the block as a way for individuals to claim additional benefits. CFS was unkindly referred to as Yuppie Flu due to the amount of people in their thirties who visited their doctors with symptoms of chronic fatigue syndrome.

The distinction between fibromyalgia syndrome and chronic fatigue syndrome rests on the fact that the former reports more joint and muscle pain while the latter reports fatigue as the major symptom. This does not mean that the two conditions mentioned have distinctly different causes. Genetic variation may account for the differences in symptoms. Indeed, genetic variation may be responsible for us looking for different causes of what is tantamount to the same disease.

In a similar vein, similar symptoms may be the result of widely differing aetiologies each amenable to quite separate treatments.

I often use the analogy that when you feel feverish, are sneezing and have a runny nose, that the two likely candidates are the common cold or an allergy. The symptoms of the common cold are the result of one of many viruses while the allergy symptoms are the result of immunoglobulin E (IgE) over-reacting to one or more allergens. These antibodies migrate to cells that release chemical causing the symptoms of intense itching, swelling and redness that are indicative of allergies.

In a cold you are quite likely to produce yellow or green mucous. This is indicative of the presence of white blood cells.

With an allergy, the mucous remains clear. However, the itching is caused by the release of histamine from mast cells.

Different processes, therefore, may lead to similar symptoms and separating them out is not always easy.

Regardless of this, these conditions – whether they are one or the same or not - impact greatly on the quality of life.

This book will explore the underlying processes which contribute to the condition known as fibromyalgia but chronic fatigue syndrome will also be explored to try and ascertain whether they are one and the same syndrome.

There continue to be many different theories surrounding these nebulous disorders but one thing cannot be discounted. They are very real conditions which deserve more recognition – and understanding - than they currently have.

I do not stand from the position of believing that these syndromes have only one cause. It is therefore important to look at possible culprits (note the plural) and either eliminate the potential culprit or add a nutrient to correct a deficiency state.

For far too long medical research has been fixated on finding one cause for a particular syndrome although comorbidities are not unusual by any stretch of the imagination.

For example, psoriasis generally accompanies psoriatic arthritis and bears a significantly increased risk of Crohn's disease, uveitis and a number of psychological and psychiatric disorders.

A thorough knowledge of existing conditions may very well point us in the direction of the cause of fibromyalgia syndrome (FMS) or chronic fatigue syndrome (CFS) since they may share metabolic pathways.

People may very firmly say that the causative factor was a virus. That may be true but debilitating illness often deprives us of nutrients. It may not be so much the virus that is at fault but that certain nutrients were used up in the battle to fight the infective agent; this at a time when we did not feel like eating anyway.

 We need to take a broader view when it comes to investigating the potential causes of any illness and not just assume that only one factor is involved in its manifestation.

Dedication

To Vanessa

Whose battle with life has been fought with great courage in the light of such little strength.

Fibromyalgia

Fibromyalgia – also called fibromyalgia syndrome (FMS) is a chronic condition that causes widespread bodily pain.

It is considered to be a novel syndrome but, in reality, it has been recognised since the 1820's as fibrositis. However, in 1976 it was classified as fibromyalgia.

There was a specific reason why the renaming took place. It reflected a new understanding of the syndrome.

 The addition of 'itis' at the end of a word implies inflammation. Originally the muscle pain felt in this complaint was thought to be due to inflammatory processes. However, advances in medicine changed this concept. The replacement of 'itis' by 'myalgia' recognised that muscle pain was a defining characteristic of FMS but also firmly put paid to any suggestion that its cause was inflammatory in nature.

In addition to generalised pain, those with fibromyalgia may have fatigue, muscle stiffness and increased sensitivity of pain.

Mood disorders and fatigue are common. As fibromyalgia is a syndrome then this means there is a collection of symptoms of which some will be applicable and others not.

When we look at this collection of symptoms some of them are quite diverse between suffers.

However, given the descriptive label of this syndrome, if you do not have muscle pain, then you must look elsewhere for a label to describe your syndrome.

Illustration of how fibromyalgia syndrome may manifest itself in different patients

Individual one suffers from:

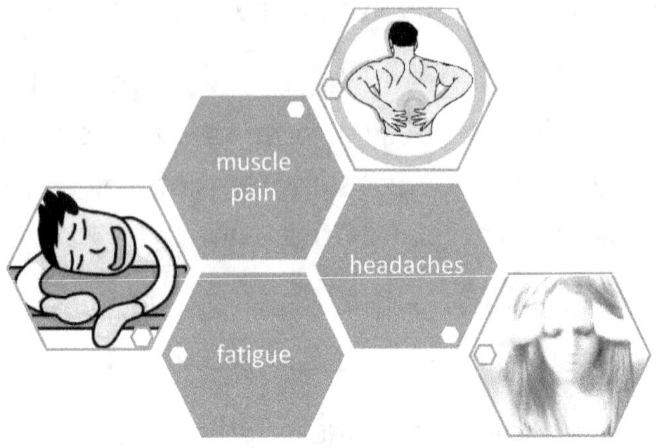

Individual two suffers from muscle pain and:

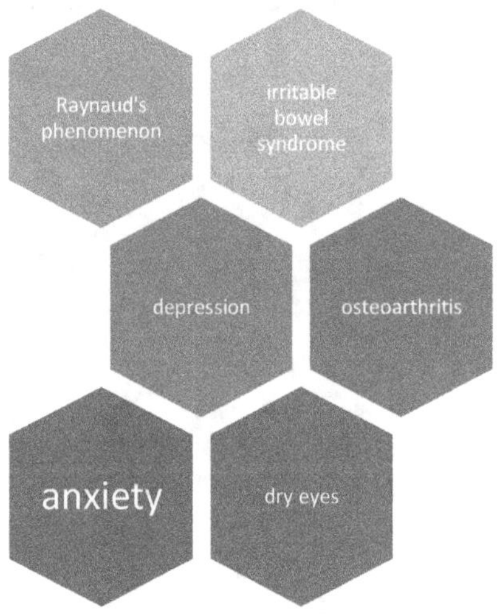

There is a wide range of symptoms characteristic of FMS. These are the most popular ones but they are not an exclusive list.

The range of symptoms found in fibromyalgia syndrome include:

- Raynaud's phenomenon (the blood vessels are overly sensitive to cold with constriction of blood vessels leading to hands which turn very white due to the lack of circulation
- Muscular pain and stiffness
- Insomnia and fatigue
- Depression and anxiety
- Irritable bowel syndrome
- Severe headaches
- Any type of arthritis
- Dry eyes and dry mouth
- Allergies, sinusitis, restless leg syndrome, sensitive bladder and angioedema

Many people suffer from muscle pain but this, by itself, is not fibromyalgia. Muscle pain has to be accompanied by painful pressure points in order for it to be diagnosed as fibromyalgia.

There are 18 tender points which are recognised as being associated with fibromyalgia syndrome. For a diagnosis to be made, the expectation is that there will be pain, on pressure, in at least eleven of them.

The pain points are bilateral and are found in:

- The inner knee
- Lower front muscles of the neck
- Outer hip
- Supraspinatus muscles in the shoulder blade area
- Trapezius muscles of the back - shoulder area
- Upper chest just beneath the collarbone
- Base of the skull at the neck area
- Outside of the elbow where the tendons attach to the bone
- Upper outer quadrant of the gluteal muscle of the buttocks

There are similarities with fibromyalgia syndrome and chronic fatigue syndrome. There are many overlapping symptoms although in fibromyalgia syndrome – as its name suggests – it has muscular pain as its dominant symptom as opposed to chronic fatigue syndrome which is mainly characterised by profound tiredness. Both of these conditions appear to follow an illness or severe emotional shock.

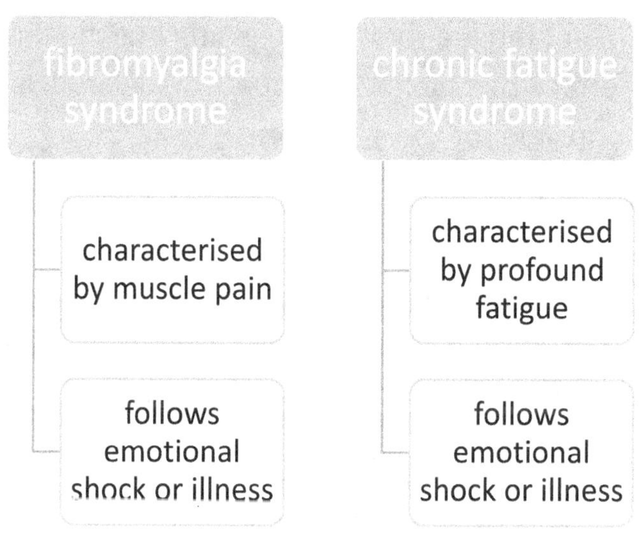

From this we can make a good guess that the stress response and an infective agent were involved initially.

The findings that fibromyalgia does not appear to be inflammatory in nature has left a conundrum which is still being explored.

It does need to be explored because chronic fatigue syndrome (CFS) and fibromyalgia syndrome (FMS) impact on the quality of millions of people's lives daily. It is not just the physical pain and fatigue that is distressing but the knock on effect of not having found a specific cause responsible for the symptoms.

While a firm cause has not been established, it opens up the way for sufferers to be challenged about whether they are inventing the symptoms in order to avoid work or receive more sympathy than is deserved. This can sometimes lead to deterioration in physical, as well as mental, health.

If we are to find information about these two conditions, which might give us a clue to their cause then clearly we need to dig a little further into possible associations with other medical conditions that FMS and CFS may have.

in addition, it is helpful if the sufferer can remember when the symptoms of FMS and CFS started. Did they, for example, start after illness or an injury?

Did all the symptoms comprising the syndrome, manifest themselves together at the same time?

Is there anything that alleviates all the symptoms simultaneously or maybe a cluster of symptoms out of the whole syndrome?

Undertaking a little investigative work will bring its own rewards. Keeping a diary of what appears to worsen - or attenuate – symptoms enables you to make links between potential cause and effect. It becomes a unique living piece of research which you can refer back to time and time again.

Associations which FMS has with other conditions.

FMS does not sit in isolation from the rest of the body. It is highly likely that it shares some features as of other conditions.

There are a number of conditions which are associated with FMS and these include:

- Irritable bowel syndrome
- Anxiety and depression
- Postural orthostatic tachycardia syndrome (POTS)
- Migraine
- Sleep disorders including restless legs syndrome
- Raynaud's phenomenon

If we look at them in more detail, we may find something which links them all.

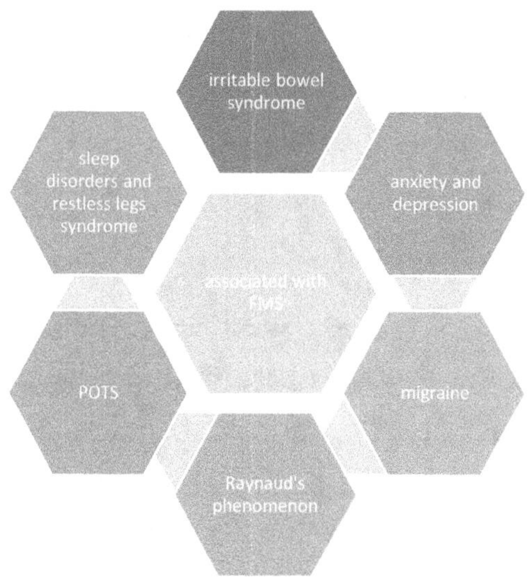

A little about each of the above conditions

1. **Irritable bowel syndrome (IBS)** – Currently, there is no clear idea of the underlying causes of IBS. However, the symptoms are: abdominal pain, constipation or diarrhoea, gas and bloating. When we look at the gut in more detail we find that it has an enteric nervous system which lies in the gut lining from oesophagus to the anus.

This miraculous structure is able to function independently of the brain through the millions of nerves which are part of it. It secretes enzymes and coordinates the propulsive efforts needed to push food along the gut. It also secretes a hormone called serotonin.

We call this gut derived serotonin (GDS) as opposed to the serotonin found in the brain which is acting as a neurotransmitter – a sender of messages in the brain. This is referred to as brain derived serotonin (BDS).

Gut serotonin has a lot of important functions. For example:

- it regulates how quickly food moves through your system. This is also referred to as the motility of your bowels.
- it has a regulatory effect and determines how sensitive your gut is to sensations like fullness when eating.
- It regulates how much fluid is secreted in your gut.

People who have IBS with constipation tend to have lower levels of serotonin and so their gut motility is reduced. Some of the functions which serotonin has are:

- It is the precursor for melatonin, the hormone which is involved in the sleep wake cycle.
- It improves mood
- It causes narrowing of the blood vessels
- There are some studies which link high blood levels of serotonin with osteoporosis.

It is immediately obvious that irritable bowel syndrome is associated with mood and sleep disorders but can it be connected to restless legs syndrome?

Well first, we need to understand what restless legs syndrome actually is.

Restless legs syndrome – this is also known as Willis-Ekbom disease.   It is a common condition of the nervous system. Sufferers experience unpleasant crawling sensations in their legs and feel an irresistable urge to move them.

No one is very sure what causes it but it is thought to be related to:

- Iron deficiency anaemia- free iron damages blood vessels
- Taking antihistamines – they cause vasoconstriction
- Taking antidepressants – increases serotonin and/or noradrenaline which cause vasoconstriction
- Lack of Magnesium – which can cause vasoconstriction
- Lack of vitamin D which can cause vasoconstriction
- Histamine can cause inflammation which can also cause restless legs. However, in this case, the blood vessels will be dilated and will irritate nerves.

Research does support the view that some cases of restless leg syndrome may be caused by a deficiency of magnesium. Magnesium reduces inflammation and pain. It also helps to dilate blood vessels.

Research has also shown a link between low vitamin D levels, restless legs syndrome and poor sleep quality. Adequate Vitamin D is required to reduce inflammation throughout the body and brain.

There are vitamin D receptors everywhere in the body including the brain. This shows just how important vitamin D is for the health of the whole body.

So, we now have an idea of what restless legs syndrome is but how is it associated with irritable bowel syndrome and more importantly fibromyalgia syndrome?

A study[1] published in NMJ online on the 9th October 2012 made the connection.

This comparative control study took 225 individuals with diagnosed IBS and 262 healthy

---

[1] https://www.ncbi.nlm.nih.gov/pmc/articles/PMC3479257/

age and sex matched controls to compare the prevalence rate of restless legs syndrome between them.

It was found that IBS was significantly associated with restless legs syndrome.

Although the underlying mechanism of IBS is unknown the association with psychological and neurological factors has been mooted.

In addition, the disruption of enteric and central nervous system communication potentially caused by inflammatory mediators triggered by bacterial overgrowth has been theorised.

Strangely, small intestinal bacterial overgrowth has been found to be connected to restless legs syndrome and fibromyalgia syndrome, too.

The syndrome, which has so often been referred to as a product of imagination appears to have valid connections.

Perhaps then one possible treatment is the restoration of good gut microbiota especially after antibiotics have been prescribed.

However, foods high in iron can also disrupt gut microbiota. Many pregnant mums who take iron tablets for the very first time, will testify to the fact that it is constipating. It may be prudent to look at why this phenomenon occurs.

Why is iron constipating?

Iron is hard on the digestive tract and frequently causes constipation. It isn't easy to absorb as it needs to have a particular charge to be absorbed by the cells of the small intestine.

Further, iron will only be absorbed in the small intestine if the iron is in its ferrous state. Ferric iron cannot be absorbed so it will travel to the colon where it is likely to cause dysbiosis (imbalance of good and bad bacteria) and subsequently, constipation.

Even when iron is absorbed in the small intestine, it needs to go through a series of reactions before it can be made available to the body.

Slow release forms of iron – which are sometimes prescribed – are not necessarily less constipating. The first part of your intestine – the jejenum and duodenum - are where the iron is absorbed best. However, slow release iron may not be released until it reaches the colon where it has the potential to cause dysbiosis.

The colon is full of bacteria that regulates the gut environment, supports bowel motility and stool quality. In other words, as we have already seen, a healthy gut biome means healthy bowel movements.

Pathogenic gut bacteria feed on iron and can upset the balance of the gut biome. *Constipation suggests that an unhealthy balance of gut bacteria exists in the colon.*

It is always recommended that an iron supplement **isn't** taken when an individual has an acute bacterial infection since the protective effects of the gut biome are compromised.

To reduce the chances of suffering from the side effects of iron, use the lowest dose possible. There are some non-constipating forms of liquid iron available. Ask your doctor to prescribe that if it is required.

Milk, calcium and antacids should not be taken at the same time as iron supplements as it reduces the absorption of iron. Taking iron supplements at the same time as the above will definitely cause the digestive problems that we are trying to avoid.

In addition, many antacids that contain calcium have a constipating effect. If you really need an antacid, then choose one that contains magnesium.

Chocolate contains iron; it is also high in fat. Chocolate is a likely cause of constipation through its ability to dysregulate gut motility. Further, fat slows down the passage of food through the intestinal tract. This can contribute to the digestive issues that we are trying to avoid.

However, the important message that needs to be taken away from this is that any foods high in iron have the potential to disrupt gut microflora as bad bacteria feed off iron.

Some foods which are high in iron are:

- Chocolate
- Red meat
- Mushrooms
- Dried fruit
- Fortified cereals
- Shellfish
- Dark leafy greens
- Beans and lentils

The recommended daily value is 18mg and it may be a useful exercise to look at your daily intake of iron for three or four days to ascertain whether this may be contributing to the problem.

In some cases, iron is necessary to avoid iron deficiency anaemia. As iron has the ability to cause IBS –C, through an imbalance of good gut bacteria, then there are a number of steps you can take that would ameliorate this.

- if iron is required use non constipating forms of liquid iron. Do not take with antacids
- reduce fat in the diet but do not eliminate it as it does help absorb fat soluble vitamins.
- Take a tablespoon of olive oil a day as this helps bowel movements. This can be used with a tablespoon of vinegar and made into a salad dressing. Vinegar is useful for preventing bloating and helps peristalsis – the movement of food along the gastrointestinal tract. Vinegar also introduces new populations of good gut bacteria into the colon.
- Use a prebiotic such as inulin powder to provide 'food' for gut bacteria. This will aid any bloating, if this is one of the more troubling symptoms of gastroparesis.
- Fermented foods help promote the growth of beneficial probiotics or good

bacteria. As such they can help with bloating but they do have mixed results on gastroparesis.

Some individuals will benefit from adding fermented foods to their diet and others won't. This would be likely due to genetic differences. Foods in vinegar, kefir, cheese and yogurt are all examples of fermented foods. However, do not take dairy foods at the same time as iron medication as they would rapidly cause discomfort.

Iron overload

The symptoms of iron overload are many but include:

- Chronic fatigue
- Joint pain
- Abdominal pain
- Osteoarthritis
- Infertility
- Elevated blood sugar
- Depression
- Migraines/headaches

In fact, many of the symptoms that form part of the syndrome that we know as FMS.

Now that we have established a connection between migraine and ibs and FMS, it is probably useful to look at migraine and its connection with these troubling syndromes. However, it would be useful at the end of this long chapter to summarise what we have learned so far.

Fibromyalgia syndrome is a collection of symptoms whose predominant feature is muscle pain.

There appears to be a gut-brain connection and although the myalgia does not immediately appear to be caused inflammation, it may be referred pain from processes going on elsewhere in the body, predominantly the gut which may have links to inflammation and/or bacterial overgrowth.

There also appears to be a link with serotonin deficiency. Serotonin levels are intimately connected with the way muscles behave. Low serotonin may cause chronic pain and it is strongly associated with FMS.

Serotonin is also necessary for gut motility so low levels can be implicated in constipation

Patients diagnosed with FMS are often given anti-depressants known as SSRI's. These raise serotonin levels. They are often effective in ameliorating many of the symptoms of this puzzling syndrome.

However, anti-depressants do not come without unwanted side effects and you may wish to try adding foods to your diet that increase serotonin levels, first. These include:

- Salmon
- Spinach
- Poultry
- Nuts and seeds
- Eggs
- Milk and cheese
- Pineapple
- Tofu and soy

Now we have brought serotonin out as a possible contributor to FMS, it draws our attention to migraine which also has an association with FMS.

Migraine

Migraineurs will tell you that this condition is probably the most debilitating and painful condition that they have ever suffered.

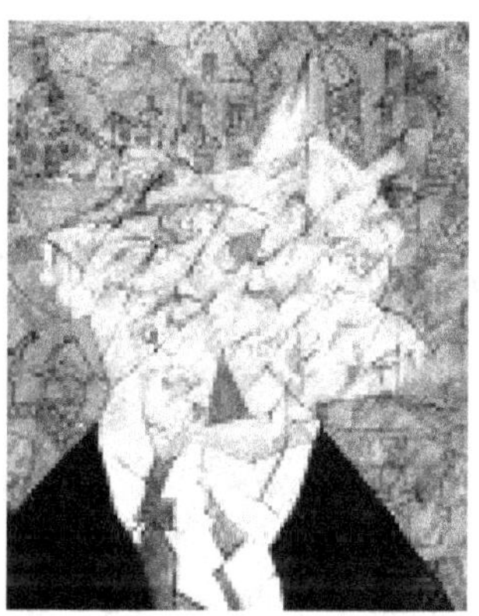

Migraine is extremely debilitating

As a former migraineur I can concur with that and I have personally experienced the nausea, vomiting and gut disturbances that go with it. The sensitivity to light and sound can only be understood by those who have experienced such violent symptoms. The pillow that was once so soft can feel as though it is filled with rocks.

To understand how migraine can fill us with such impending doom is better explained by understanding the stages that it goes through and what underpins them.

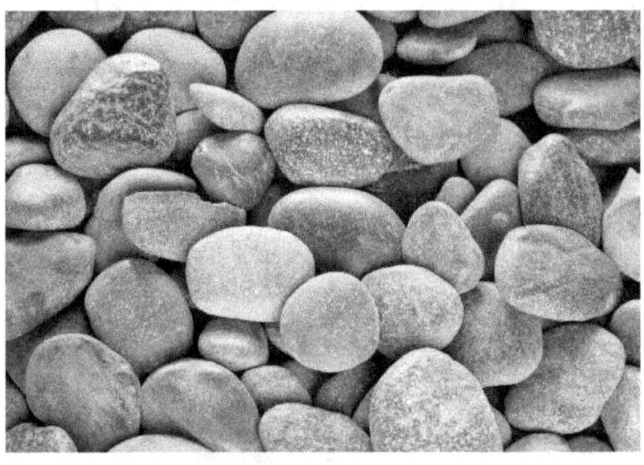

Having migraine feels like sleeping on a pillow full of rocks

The pattern of events in migraine is:

spreading depression – loss of activity in groups of nerve cells in the brain (aura stage)
Reduced blood flow through blood vessels
Relaxation of blood vessels and damage to nerve endings. This stimulation will cause pain.
Formation and release of a number of inflammatory mediators causing tissue damage and increased pain caused by the extra stretching on nerve endings in dilated blood vessels
The leakiness is further increased so that more substances involved in leakiness can gain access to the blood vessel increasing the pain even further.

The reduced blood flow seen in the blood vessels at the initial stages of the condition is due to serotonin which constricts the blood flow. Serotonin is able to dilate and constrict blood vessels depending on prevailing influences.

This stage is followed by the relaxed stage where the dilation of the blood vessels stretches and damages the nerve endings. This will cause pain and tissue damage.

When tissue damage occurs then inflammatory substances pour into the damaged areas causing leakiness and pain.

The sympathetic nervous system is responsible for the diameter of the blood vessels. At rest, sympathetic nerves will constrict the arterioles in muscle. However, exercise can cause epinephrine to act on beta 2 receptors. This can cause blood vessels to widen.

There is a condition known as abdominal migraine which is poorly understood. It is found in children and those who suffer from it will eventually morph into the migraine/headache only type.

Nevertheless, they share similar triggers such as:

- exposure to light and sound
- poor sleep
- foods containing chocolate (one of my triggers)
- monosodium glutamate (MSG)
- skipping meals

Studies have shown that when MSG and aspartame are taken together, then levels of serotonin are reduced.

Although most people will be familiar with the concept that MSG is connected to Chinese food, they may not know that aspartame is found in:

- frozen desserts
- gelatine
- cereals
- soft drinks including diet ones
- milk drinks
- sugar free chewing gum
- tea and instant coffee

If you are particularly fond of chinese cuisine, it may be prudent to avoid foods containing aspartame to see if it reduces the symptoms of fibromyalgia.

Some people do appear to have twitchy blood vessels which respond to very slight changes in the environment and which would not bother the majority of the populate.

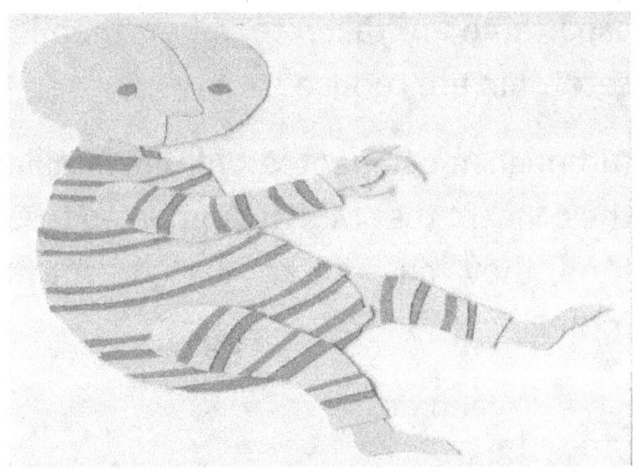

Some people have especially twitchy blood vessels

Neurotransmitter profiles are also subject to genetic variation and environmental factors and more than adequately explain why one person suffers from FMS and others do not.

Raynaud's phenomenon

Many people who are eventually diagnosed with autoimmune disease find that one of their first symptoms is Raynaud's phenomenon. It's appearance may occur years before other symptoms manifest themselves enough for the patient to take themselves off to the doctor for diagnosis.

Raynaud's phenomenon occurs when the small blood vessels in the extremities - such as the hands or feet - are over sensitive to tiny changes in temperature. Stress is also implicated.

Although most people are plagued with Raynaud's in the winter, I recall having bouts of it during a very hot summer. I had cut my food intake down a great deal due to the heat and can only assume that this was the cause. Certainly, in my much younger days such an action would have resulted in the onset of a migraine within a couple of hours.

 The extremities involved in Raynaud's phenomenon turn red before appearing almost bloodless as the tiny blood vessels constrict in protest at the temperature change.

It is an exquisitely painful condition and can make fine tasks - like buttoning up a shirt - impossible.

The culprit in this condition appears to be a neurotransmitter called norepinephrine (noradrenaline) which constricts blood vessels.

Now serotonin has a bit of a Jekyll and Hyde nature. It can cause blood vessels to constrict and it can cause them to dilate. Sometimes, it helps to potentiate the effects of other vaso constrictors like norepinephrine so we have not quite lost that serotonin connection just yet.

Alpha 1 blockers can counter the effect of norepinephrine but these blockers do not have to be prescribed medication.

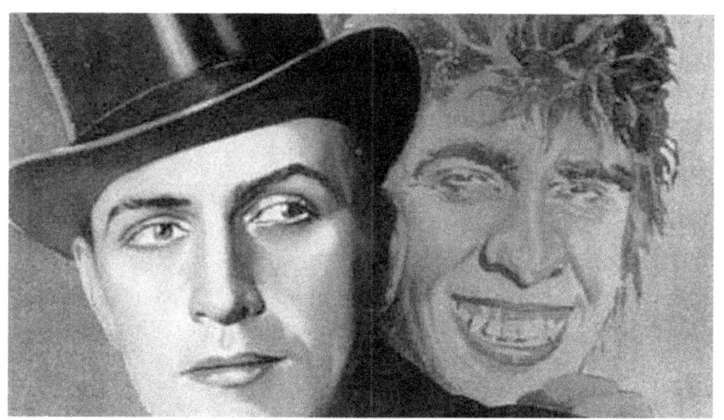

Serotonin has a Jekyll and Hyde character

Alpha 1 blockers are found in a number of foods and these include:

- L-arginine, an amino acid, is a natural alpha blocker and is found in all meat, nuts and seeds and leafy vegetables.
- Foods containing potassium such as tomatoes
- Garlic
- Coenzyme Q10
- Foods containing magnesium which include beans, nuts and fish are good sources.

As an aside, although I used to have migraine and Raynaud's on a regular basis I no longer have these episodes. I suspect diet changes have helped but the underlying susceptibility will always be there.

Postural Tachycardia Syndrome (PoTS).

It is not surprising that we have yet another collection of symptoms packaged together as a syndrome which aptly describes its features if not the underlying aetiology.

 This syndrome occurs when there is a rapid and abnormal increase in heart rate that occurs after sitting or standing. Individuals will feel dizzy and, in some cases, faint when rising from a position.

POTS occurs because when you sit or stand up, gravity will cause some of your blood to pulled to your extremities.   Normally, your blood vessels will respond to this change of position by narrowing blood vessels and increasing heart rate. This helps to maintain the blood flow to the heart and brain. In addition, it prevents blood pressure dropping.

 in POTS, the autonomic nervous system (ANS) does not work properly. The blood vessels do not narrow as they should and there is a drop in blood supply to the brain and heart when you become upright.   The heart increases its pumping to compensate for this – hence the tachycardia which partially describes this syndrome.

This excessive rise in heart rate is accomplished through an increase of norepinephrine into the blood stream which is orchestrated by serotonin.

Anxiety and depression

Most people will, at some point in their lives, suffer from anxiety and depression. For many, it may be a temporary reaction to external events that overwhelm them until we adjust or work through them.

Others may find that anxiety and depression have dogged them throughout their lives. Whether it is lack of coping mechanisms, social support or some genetic flaw may not be clear. What is clear is that mental health has a far reaching impact on relationships, physical health and life choices.

The underlying mechanisms to anxiety and depression are well established. When acute stress occurs, the body's sympathetic nervous system in activated by the sudden release of hormones.

The sympathetic nervous system brings about actions that aren't under our voluntary control.

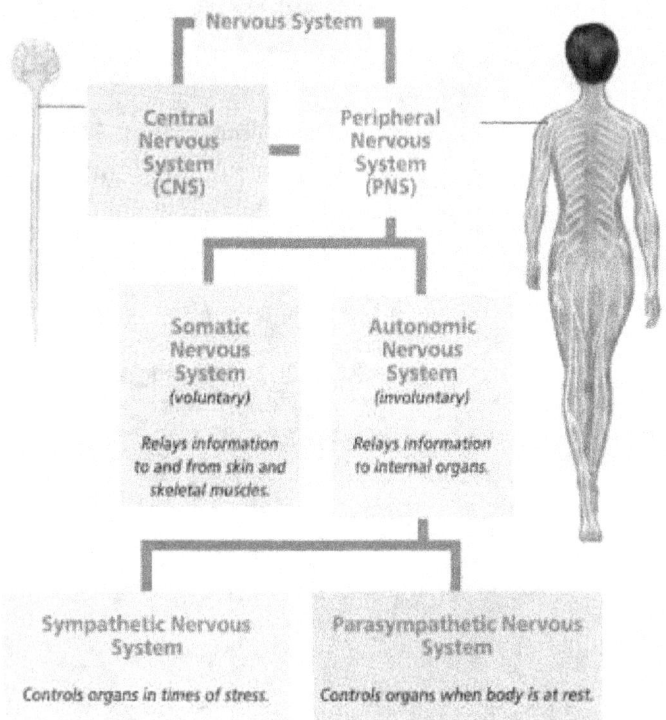

The function of the sympathetic nervous system only occurs through the connection of the internal organs to the brain by the spinal nerves.

These nerves need to be stimulated before preparing the organism for action. It does this by increasing the heart rate, increasing blood flow to the muscles while simultaneously decreasing blood flow to the skin. The latter would happen in Raynaud's as we have discussed earlier. .

 Initially, in this stress response, the adrenal glands – which sit on top of the kidneys – are activated and trigger the release of cortisol.

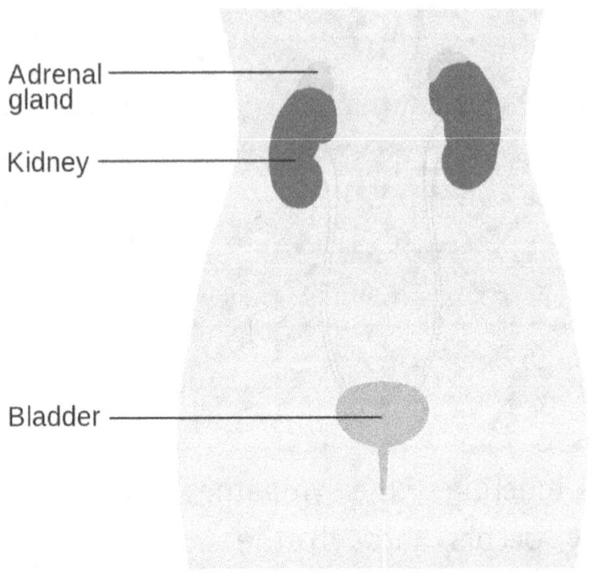

Cortisol is a hormone that plays an important role in many bodily functions including the regulation of blood pressure, the functioning of the immune system and how the body uses glucose. For example, when you have an infectious disease the immune system is geared up to fight the infection by cortisol secretion. Once extra cortisol is not required your body will return to a state of relaxation.

Nevertheless, if cortisol production is continuous or prolonged as a result of stress, then high blood sugar, high blood pressure and a reduced ability to fight infections occurs. It also causes fat to be stored in the body. These symptoms are not unlike those found in metabolic syndrome.

The symptoms of high cortisol are similar to those of FMS. They include:

- Irritability
- Anxiety and depression
- Fatigue
- Headaches
- Increased blood pressure
- Symptoms of IBS
- Weight gain
- Insomnia
- Difficulty recovering from exercise

However, although muscle breakdown and muscle weakness are symptoms of high cortisol. Muscle pain is not – that is more of the domain of low serotonin levels.

Over time prolonged cortisol also impacts on the appearance of your skin.

When cortisol is raised, more of the circulating blood is diverted to the organs which will be needed to play a part in the fight or flight response. Thus, blood is diverted to the heart, brain, lungs and kidneys. Less is sent to the skin.

People under prolonged stress often look tired, white and drained. Cortisol robs people of the pink tinge that people have on their cheeks when they are in good health.

As cortisol and muscle tension tend to go hand in hand, prolonged stress can also induce wrinkles. Eventually, the impact of stress can permanently settle itself into people's faces.

People under prolonged stress are generally (but not always)

- Overweight with abdominal fat and rounded cheeks
- Have tight, drawn skin which is white and unhealthy looking

Effects of Cortisol

Urge to pass urine/empty bowels – this is part of the stress response which makes sure that our bladder and bowels are empty before we start fighting otherwise we would be at a distinct disadvantage to our enemies.

Tremor and sweating - normally we sweat in response to external heat sources or physical activity. This is produced by eccrine glands.

The sweat from stress is not a heat sweat and is produced by your apocrine glands. The tremor is also a result of the revved up responses going on in your body.

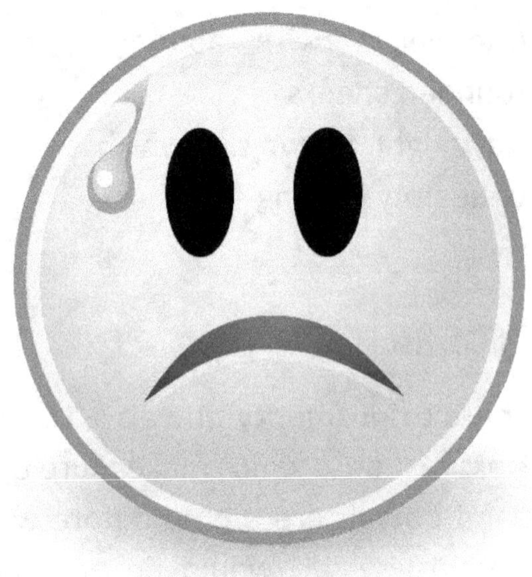

The sweat from stress is produced by apocrine glands which are different from the glands that produce a heat sweat.

Pins and needles – this is due to an active stress response. The cortisol diverts blood to vital organs. Those which aren't vital will constrict and tighten which can give rise to the feeling of pins and needles.

The psychological symptoms of anxiety are

- Agitation
- Tension

- Irritability
- A feeling of being detached
- Fear of losing control of the situation
- A feeling of impending doom

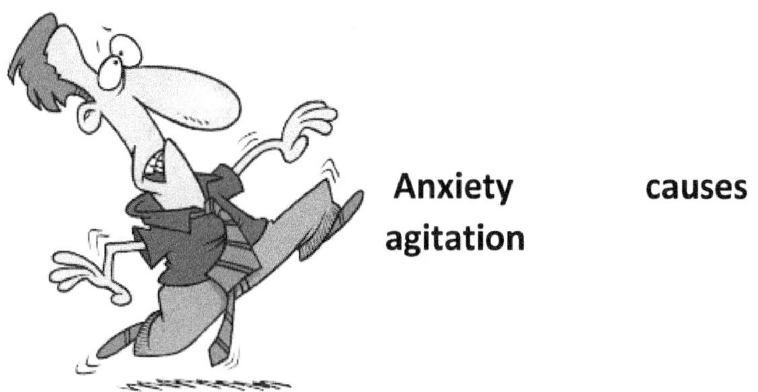

Anxiety causes agitation

Treatment for depression normally involves talking therapies such as CBT and/or medication such as selective serotonin reuptake inhibitors also known as SSRI's.

Serotonin is made from an amino acid called tryptophan which is found in carbohydrates. This is why people who are feeling stressed have a tendency to eat a high carbohydrate diet. It has a calming effect.

Antidepressants such as sertraline – one of the SSRI's - can be taken long term but a low dose will be started on first before being increased gradually.

The downside to SSRI's is that they do not appear to be effective for a number of weeks. Further, they can have quite a number of unwanted sided effects such as:

- Feeling or being sick
- Diarrhoea or constipation
- Loss of weight
- Indigestion
- Insomnia
- Excessive sweating
- Headaches
- Erectile dysfunction

If the SSRI's aren't effective. then a serotonin and noradrenaline reuptake inhibitor (SNRI's) may be prescribed. This type of medicine increases the amount of serotonin and noradrenaline in your brain.

The general function of noradrenaline is to get the brain and body ready for action. The amount of noradrenaline synthesised is at its lowest during sleep and at its highest during situations which involve the flight or fight response.

In the brain, noradrenaline increases arousal and alertness. It helps memory and helps focus attention.

It can also cause anxiety and restlessness. Anxiety is extremely distressing. Anything which is likely to increase anxiety needs to be considered carefully.

Further undesirable side effects of noradrenaline   include an increase in heart rate and blood pressure. Blood flow to the gastrointestinal system is reduced. It can also cause constipation.

 Just like SSRI's, SNRI's also have some nasty side effects. In fact, anxious people are likely to be made even more anxious by the side effects.

Pulling everything together

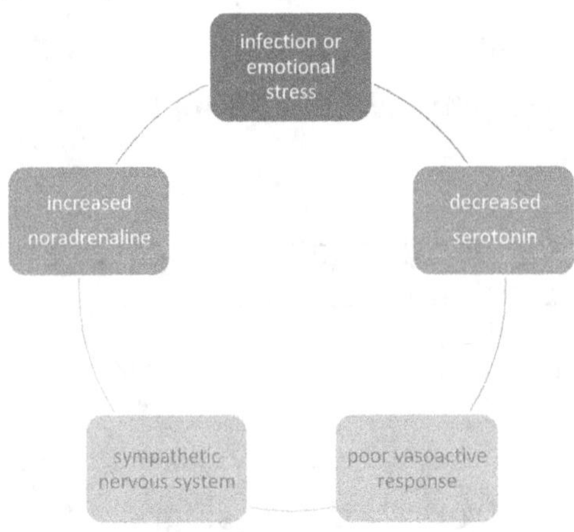

Infection or emotional stress do impact levels of serotonin and noradrenaline

The sympathetic nervous system's main function is to keep many of the processes in the body functioning and in harmony with other processes. It is, for example responsible for:

- Gut motility
- Urinary system output and function

- Fight or flight syndrome
- vasoconstriction

among many others.

Many of the FMS related conditions appear to be related to the sympathetic nervous system which is responsible for, among others, the state of our blood vessels which appear to be overly sensitive to triggers especially stress.

However, we have also mentioned that infection can impact these two hormones.

However, right at the beginning of this book I stated that the renaming of fibrositis to fibromyalgia occurred because inflammation was not found around the tender muscle points which are used to diagnose FMS.

However, there are a number of reasons why the muscles may not have looked hot and swollen as you would expect if inflammation or infection had been present.

These include:

- referred pain – that is there was an injury or infection elsewhere and the pain was transmitted to the joints and surrounding areas. This happens quite a lot. For example, kidney pain is often felt around the shoulder blade.
- it could be a pain memory from a previous illness such as influenza.
- Pain, regardless of where the injury is is actually perceived in the brain. Maybe there are pockets of inflammation or infection in the brain that are contributing to the pain elsewhere.

When we consider the joint and muscle pain which is felt in FMS then the inflammatory mediator which comes to mind is the mast cell. This generally resides around connective tissue and could account for the pain felt as part of the myalgia.

However, there are a great many mast cells to be found around joints, stomach, intestines and skin, among other sites which could be

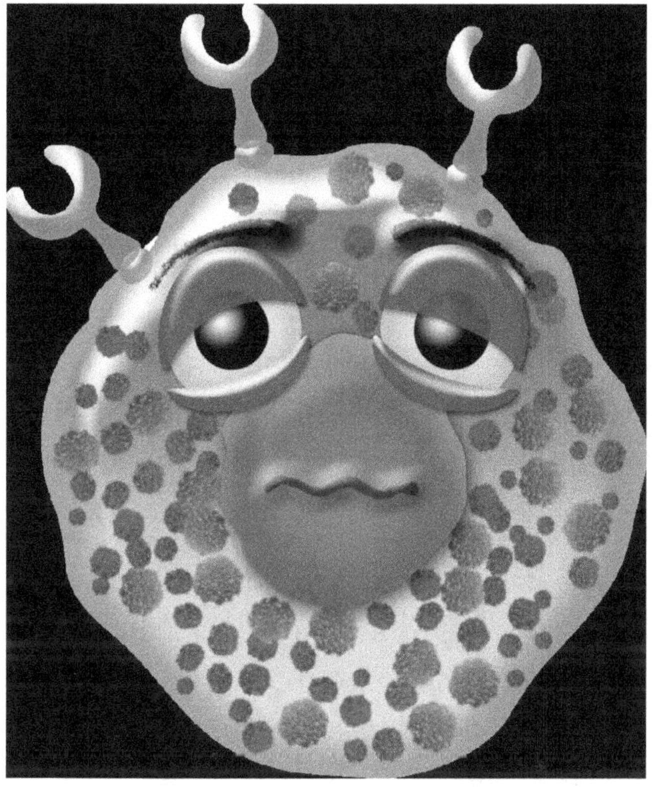

Mast cells contain histamine which makes blood vessels leaky and allows others cells of the immune system to squeeze through.

Significant in our search for answers to FMS.

Mast cells contain histamine. Mast cells release histamine into areas that need greater access by other immune system cells as a response to injury or infection. Histamine helps immune cells get to where they need to go by making them leaky and open.

 The ensuing dilation of blood vessels stretches nerve endings and this creates pain. This is part of the process that happens in those who suffer from the excruciating pain of migraine.

Histamine deserves examination. Firstly, its effects are systemic. Excessive histamine - or an intolerance to histamine - can make you feel very ill indeed.

 Histamine has a similar effect to prostaglandins. It has an important role in the early inflammatory response and is therefore most associated with acute inflammation. Nevertheless, it is to a lesser degree implicated in chronic pain.

As histamine's actions are not localised, it can cause widespread pain.

There is condition known as histamine intolerance. It has a myriad of symptoms including:

- pain associated with inflammation as normally found in rheumatic diseases or rheumatoid arthritis such as knuckle joint rheumatism.
- soft tissue rheumatism, for example; this includes pain in the tendons, joints, back pain. Studies show that soft tissue rheumatism feels like a strained muscle or muscle ache.

The Marion institute stated that histamine could be responsible for muscular rheumatism or inflammation of a muscle.[2]as well as the above mentioned candidates.

People with histamine intolerance tend to feel very ill, very often. The see saw nature of the manifestation of their condition would be

---

[2] https://www.marioninstitute.org/histamine-intolerance-syndrome/

driven by foods that are eaten as part of the daily diet.

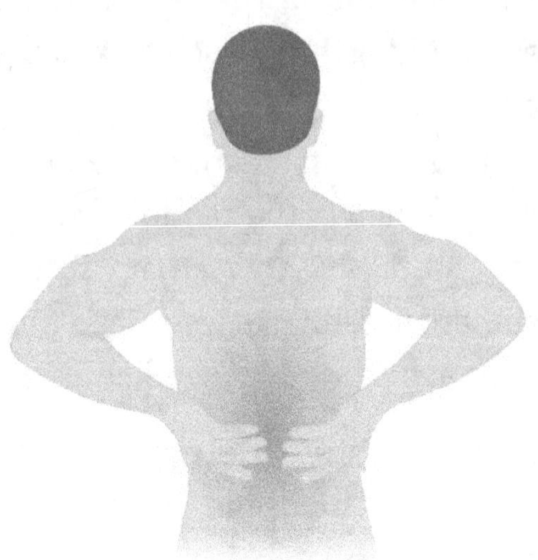

Histamine causes muscle and joint pain

The effects of histamine are much more widespread than the above picture illustrates. Nevertheless, it serves as a useful reminder that muscle aches may have nothing to do with any injury to the muscle.

 Histamine intolerance can make you feel truly awful.

The best way to counteract the effects of histamine intolerance is to go on a low histamine diet.

Histamine is found in many foods nowadays such as

- tomato ketchup
- fermented foods
- anything pickled
- cured or fermented meats
- wine beer alcohol
- tomatoes, aubergine, spinach
- canned fish

Many of these foods are more in use nowadays than they were in the past. This could account, in some respects for the rise in cases of FMS.

It is quite difficult to avoid foods containing histamine but fresh foods will contain less histamine than if they have been stored for a couple of days before being eaten.

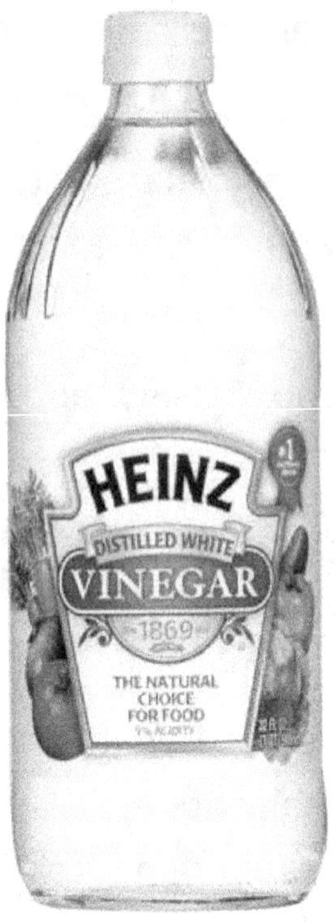

Vinegar contains histamine

Of course antihistamines are an effective treatment for histamine intolerance.

Antihistamines work very well in many types of chronic pain which is unrelated to the allergies that they are so often associated with.

If you have joint pain it is well worth trying an antihistamine[3] if you cannot tolerate NSAID's which are generally prescribed for pain.

NSAID's such as ibuprofen have been found not to work for those who have FMS so an alternative analgesic is useful.

Professor Theoharis Theorharides of Tufts University found that two drugs used in treating pain –amytriptyline and doxepin elixir – just happened to have histamine reducing properties.

Diamine oxidase (DAO) is the major enzyme involved in histamine metabolism. It ensures that there is the correct level of histamine available required for the balance of numerous chemical reactions taking place in the body.

---

[3] Vitamin C is an excellent natural antihistamine. Olive oil balances histamine.

DAO also degrades any extracellular (free) histamine which might have occurred through diet or from allergy induced processes in the body.

Olive oil has been found to release DAO into the bloodstream by up to 500%[4]

Reducing histamine may make you a little less alert so antihistamines are better taken at night. They are generally one dose daily although there are shorter acting ones such as the well-known Piriton.

Like any medication, it is for short term use only until the cause has been addressed – preferably through changes in diet and lifestyle.

Vitamin C is well known for acting in an antihistamine like way. Blood histamine levels seem to be inversely associated with the amount

---

[4] Wollin, A, wang, X, Tso, P. (2017) Nutrients regulate diamine oxidase release from intestinal mucosa). The American Physiological Society, 20, 220

of circulating vitamin C so that the greater the vitamin C the less histamine there will be.

 In some respects, vitamin C could act as a sleep aid for those with histamine induced insomnia found in FMS.

Vitamin C, like vitamin B6, is a cofactor of DAO and so sufficient intake of these vitamins is required to make DAO.

Vitamin C is found in fresh fruit and vegetables. It is easily destroyed by cooking and sunlight.

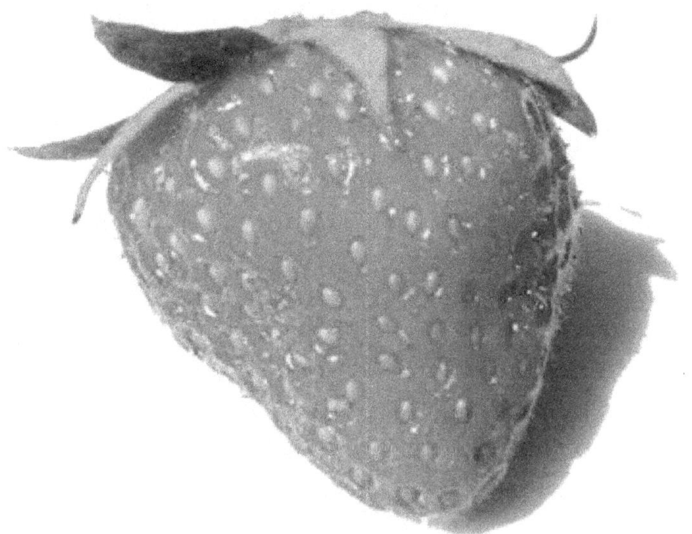

There is plenty of vitamin C in fruit.

Vitamin B6 is found in meat, nuts and whole grains.

Zinc is a marvellous trace mineral which is required for so many actions in the body that it deserves more recognition than it gets.

More than 2800 macromolecules require zinc as part of their composition. Over 300 enzymes require zinc in order to be synthesised.

My cousin who had some wart like lumps on his arm that he couldn't get rid of no matter what he used was placed on a course of zinc for insulin resistance.

Within 3 weeks, all but the largest lump had dried up and dropped off and the remaining one – which had been an open lesion – had reduced to half its size and was no longer an open lesion.

It is also worth mentioning that his beard started to grow back black even though it had been white and fairly fine for twenty years.

Zinc also prevents the release of histamine from mast cells. Now, most people can quote that vitamin C - and even quercetin - is effective against histamine but I have never heard anyone say, 'I have a histamine intolerance so I will take more zinc.'

Most people are zinc deficient. This may be surprising given the array of foods that it is found in. However, as veganism and vegetarianism become more popular there is an increased risk of zinc deficiency. The phytates that are present in vegetables bind to zinc so that the body cannot use it.

 Only a day's worth of zinc can be stored in the body and it is easily lost in urine especially if diuretics are taken.

Good sources of zinc are:

- Meat
- Fish, especially shellfish
- Dairy
- Eggs
- wholegrains
- Shellfish

Another of the symptoms of FMS can also be explained by histamine intolerance. Histamine prevents the synthesis of melatonin. Melatonin is a hormone which regulates the sleep wake cycle.

Histamine is a vasoactive substance. It also promotes the release of serotonin – another vasoactive substance - which at large concentrations causes vasodilation, like histamine.

If you eat foods which are high in histamine, then you may find dropping off to sleep – or staying asleep - difficult.

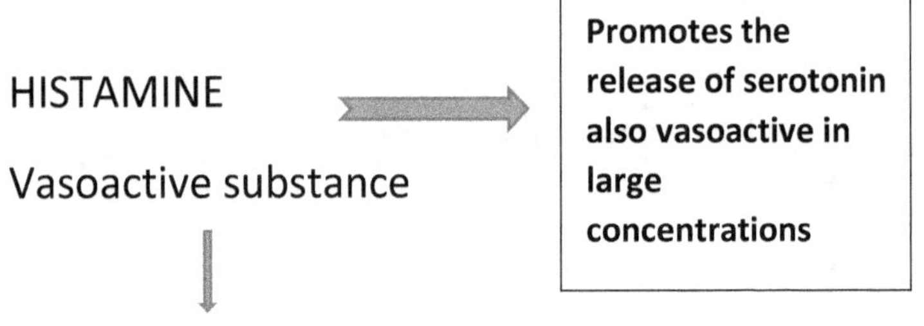

Histamine and serotonin work immediately when faced with infection or injury. They are short-lived in action and their role is to:

- increase vascular permeability
- dilate the blood vessels
- contract smooth muscle.

While these vasoactive substances may, under normal circumstances, be short-lived in their effect, a histamine intolerance can be present permanently if foods high in histamine are eaten on a regular and daily basis.

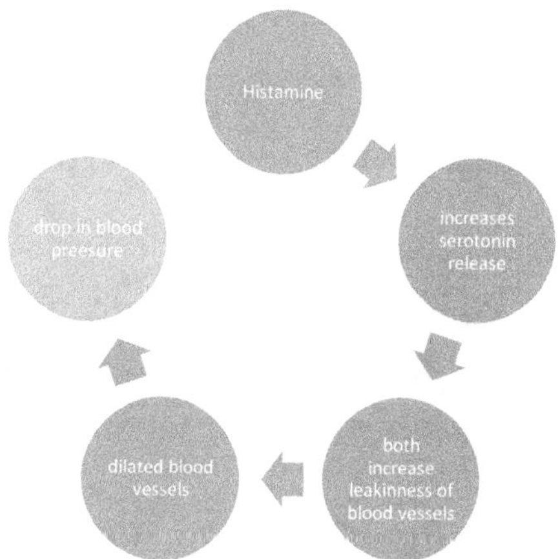

When histamine is released, common symptoms that occur are allergies (hay fever, urticaria, wheezing, for example), insomnia, pain, low blood pressure, brain fog, muscular pain, headache, brain fog, among many other symptoms.

These signs and symptoms should be vaguely familiar in that they are associated with FMS or CFS.

Histamine has its uses. It helps us learn. It keeps us alert but it also creates a leaky gut and that creates problems.

A leaky gut allows undigested food particles to enter the bloodstream. The body reacts to them as though they are foreign particle by alerting the immune system to them – particularly mast cells.

When mast cells release their contents into the bowel, symptoms of irritable bowel syndrome occur.

Histamine also provokes the release of Substance P.

Substance P is a pain transmitting chemical. It is released from the ends of specific sensory nerves and is found in the central and peripheral nervous system. It is associated with inflammatory processes and pain.

Neuronal substance P is stored in vesicles and released when it comes into contact with
- leukotrienes
- prostaglandins
- histamine

Ginger blocks both the production of prostaglandins and leukotrienes.

 In cell based studies capsaicin (found in peppers) and curcumin both blocked the production of leukotrienes.

Ibuprofen blocks prostaglandins.

Antihistamines block histamine release.

A bi directional effect is found with substance P and histamine with an increase in one raising the levels of the other.

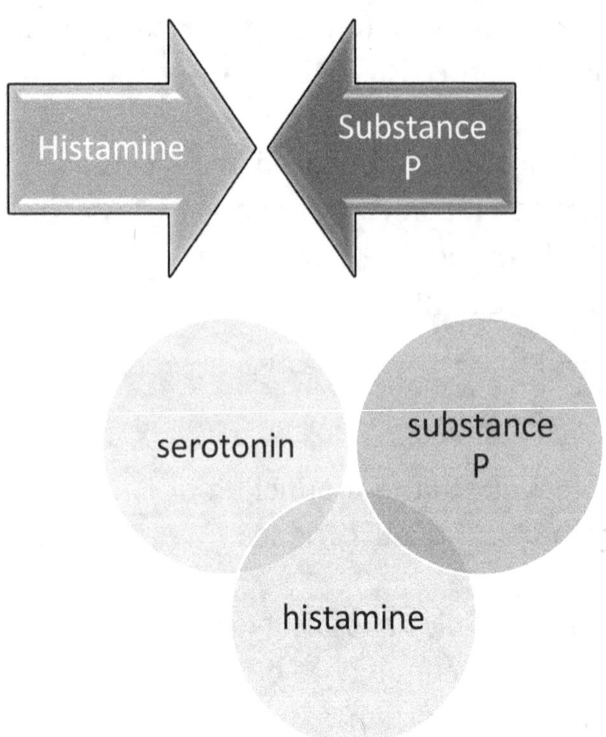

The three main contenders for the pain found in FMS.

As substance P is an interesting character, it is probably worth learning a little more of what it does.

Substance P is a pain transmitting chemical. It is released from the ends of specific sensory nerves and is found in the central and peripheral nervous system. Therefore, its potential to cause pain is widespread.

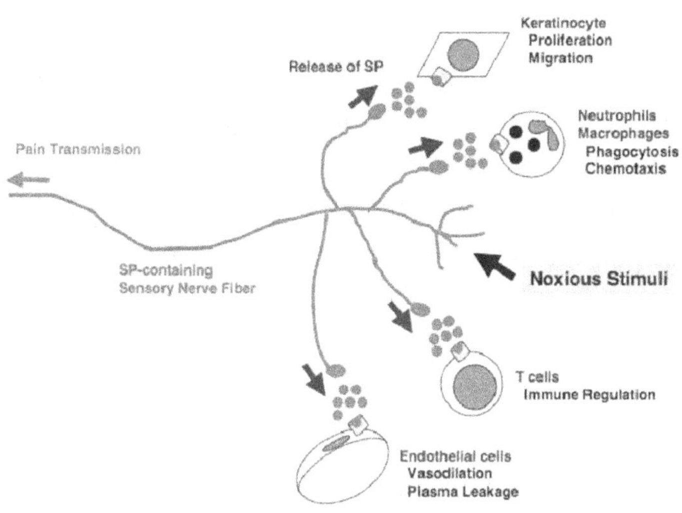

5

The nerve endings above come into contact with a noxious stimulus.   For example, a chemical irritant, cold or heat and transfer it to

---

5 https://www.researchgate.net/figure/Scheme-of-biological-functions-of-substance-P-Once-the-nerve-ending-catch-noxious_fig12_221917605

a Substance P containing nerve fibre. Substance P is capable of transmitting pain (green arrow).

It can also bind to a wide variety of immune system cells and enable them to carry out a wide range of functions.

Substance P is increased in stressful situations which promote anxiety. In addition, Substance P activates the release of histamine.

Further, stimuli like pain and heat can initiate the release of Substance P from sensory nerve endings which is proportional to the intensity of the stimuli.

It can be seen that as Substance P is associated with inflammatory processes, pain and inflammation can enhance its expression. Such activation appears to become a vicious circle where Substance P is activated by illness or injury which activates histamine.

The resultant pain induces the release of even more Substance P and further pain.

Substance P containing nerves are found in abundance at mucosal sites such as the airway. They are also found in the spinal cord, brain, the skin and around blood vessels. Substance P helps to transmit pain signals to the brain and spinal cord where pain is actually felt.

Studies have found that a nerve injury can cause a huge release of Substance P.

The release may be five-fold of that found in acute pain.

Substance P then diffuses into the surrounding area contributing to persistent pain which is characteristic of FMS.

In spite of its association with persistent pain, Substance P was found to stimulate the growth of nerve stem cells of adult rats under both normal conditions and during injury. Therefore, it could help with nerve cell formation after injury.

Neuronal substance P is stored in vesicles and released when it comes into contact with

- leukotrienes – which are also involved in the inflammatory response
- prostaglandins
- histamine

It should be clear now that Substance P is the main pain messenger in the brain. It turns up the volume of pain. It has five main areas in which it functions in the body and these are in the realm of:

- Pain
- Inflammation
- Anxiety
- Depression
- Nausea

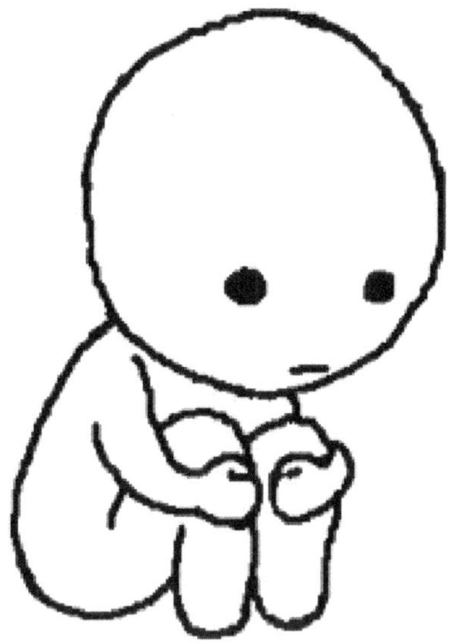

Substance P can cause depression

When too much Substance P is produced then depression can ensue but it is still a vital product. Without it, many cells of the immune system would not be called to action that is so necessary for healing of an injury to take place.

Problems only occur when there is excessive production and release of it so learning how we can keep it in check is important.

Ginger blocks both the production of prostaglandins and leukotrienes as well as Substance P.

In cell based studies capsaicin (found in peppers) and curcumin both blocked the production of leukotrienes.

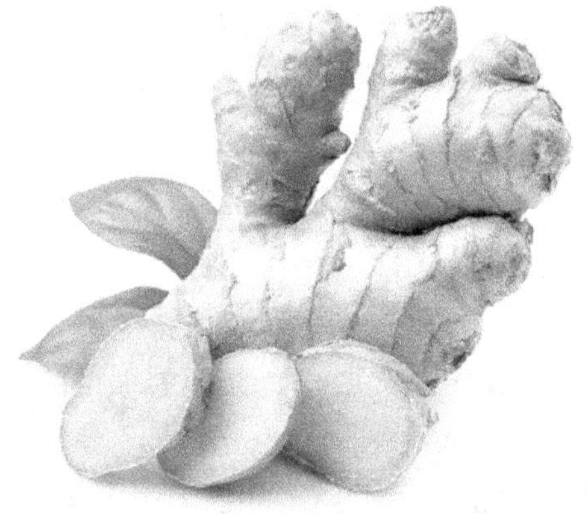

6

6

https://www.google.com/search?q=ginger&rlz=1C1GCEA_enGB828
GB828&source=lnms&tbm=isch&sa=X&ved=0ahUKEwix0Kad_cLfAh
WVrHEKHcO4BugQ_AUIDigB&biw=1366&bih=657#imgrc=M6QYox
1dER0mRM:

Although the inflammatory processes caused by Substance P - and the subsequent pain - can be addressed by over the counter medications (with an anti-inflammatory action like ibuprofen or other NSAID's), it is far better to learn how to use food as a medicine.

In many respects, histamine intolerance, given its systemic effects, fits the bill for explaining the symptoms of FMS.

 It works with other substances which increase pain and appear to be self-perpetuating.

The default pathway in FMS

Whenever pain occurs, there is a corresponding pathway formed in the brain. At first the pathway is nebulous. It has the ability to fade provided what is initiating the pain is only temporary.

 If pain continues over a long time or is intense in nature, then the pathway to pain becomes

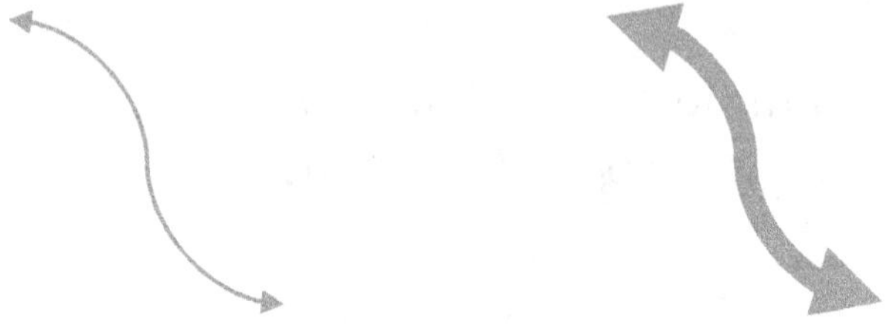

1) Pain pathway of a minor injury   2) intense pain pathway

 quite deeply etched. It becomes a default pathway where even the slightest stimulus will set it off.

We can see how the theory of pain holding pathways can play a part in the pain felt in FMS

Following a viral infection, neurological pathways are laid down in the brain. These pathways have registered the pain of muscle aches and joint pain which occur as the result of the immune response. In influenza, the pain can be quite intense and it is entirely plausible that it has been 'caught' and remembered.

Pathways in the brain are the physical representation of what we have learned. Every time we learn anything – not just pain – a pathway connecting information will form in your brain. If the event which has been 'learned' has been intense in terms of

- Severity
- Length

then the pathway is ingrained deeply and is hard to fade.

Difficulties also arise if the pathway is connected to a lot of triggers. For example, being ill can be connected to the smell of antiseptic or food. It can be connected to   certain textures such as that of the sheets. It can be associated with certain sounds such as the opening of a medicine bottle. All of these can trigger the memory of the pain felt during the illness.

Let us make no mistake, the pain that is felt is very real.

A common example is that of phantom limb pain. An amputee can still feel the pain in an amputated limb.

As I have already discussed pain registers itself in the central nervous system or spinal cord.

The timely prevention or attenuation of pain can help stop deeply etched pathways from forming a trigger happy default pathway.

Inflammation of the Central Nervous System may be a contender for FMS

More recent studies[7] using PET brain imaging have shown that glial cells are activated in the brains of patients with fibromyalgia.

Glial cells are immune system cells which are found in the brain. They do not conduct electrical signals in the way that neurons do. Instead, the glial cells surround the neurons and provide the insulation between them.

There are more glial cells in the central nervous system than there are any other type of cell.

Professor Eva Kosek and her research group found   high levels   of cytokines (substances which send messages in the brain) in the cerebrospinal fluid of individuals with FMS.

---

[7] https://ki.se/en/people/evakos

Cytokines are involved in inflammation. There are a number of these diverse, small proteins that are involved in signalling to other cells and effect how they respond.

When these cytokines are elevated then it suggests that there is an inflammatory process going on in the brain.

These findings were verified by other researchers. However, the source of the inflammation was not discovered.

The more recent use of Positron-emission topography found that the glial cells were activated and this was the cause of the inflammation. This means that glial cells are involved in the pathogenesis of FMS.

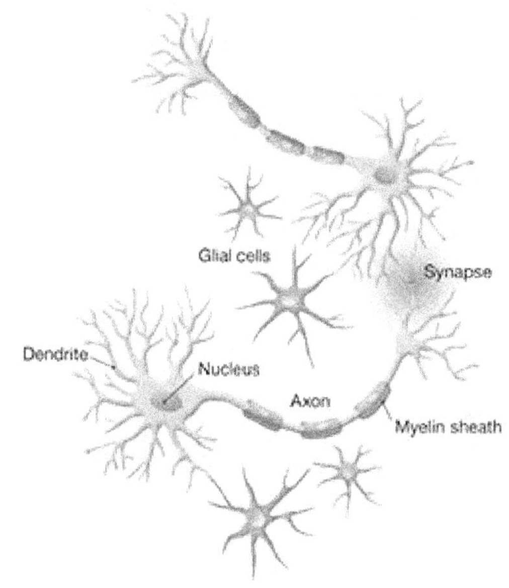

Glial cells supporting neurons.

The results also showed that the degree of inflammation correlated with the amount of fatigue felt in the participants in the study.

Now, histamine is a necessary neurotransmitter, it helps learning and memory but it is also known to cause neuroinflammation. Indeed, it is implicated in such degenerative conditions as:

- Multiple sclerosis
- Alzheimer's disease

Neuronal histamine is also implicated in pain perception to the extent that if medication is given - which increases central nervous system or peripheral nervous system (spinal cord) histamine - then medication which has an analgesic effect is given at the same time. This illustrates well histamine's ability to increase pain perception.

As we have already seen though, histamine's effect is general – there are receptors for histamine throughout the body and brain so a histamine intolerance, or imbalance or reaction to an injury or infection, can be widespread.

It accounts for all the symptoms and comorbid conditions which accompany FMS.

Further, histamine does not necessarily achieve these wide ranging symptoms by itself.

Histamine provokes two other main substances – serotonin and Substance P – to intensify pain perception. Substance P transmits pain signals to the central nervous system very efficiently.

It can be seen though, that pain relieving medication is not going to work effectively until the underlying cause of the problem is dealt with. As histamine provokes the release of serotonin and Substance P, then clearly histamine has to be dealt with before a vicious cycle of inflammation and pain is set up.

This can be achieved by:

- A low histamine diet
- Increasing DAO – the enzyme which effectively metabolises histamine
- Taking antihistamines.

This should stop the vicious cycle which has been set up.

However, I am not in favour of taking antihistamines for a prolonged period. They are good for short term use but still have side effects – both long and short – that we would wish to avoid.

They can contribute to fatigue, constipation, an ability to think properly, drowsiness. In fact, many of the symptoms that those with FMS complain about in the first place.

This diverse set of symptoms which are part of the FMS syndrome are not unusual and are mainly down to genetic differences.

Nevertheless, as we have seen, the underlying instigator of the cause of FMS – can be various infections or injury. As these can have different symptoms – influenza feels different from viral meningitis -this will result in the wide range of symptoms – that are characteristic of FMS. An individual's experience of whichever infective agent they encountered will have been recorded in the neurological pathways which register pain.

In addition, the individual will have been influenced by different environmental experiences. When ill, patients may be looked after in hospital or tended at home, for example.

These experiences will engender their own unique set of triggers which are specific to each individual. We perhaps do not always appreciate how many details of our lives are stored in the brain or for how long. I have only to smell cigarette smoke to be transported to a scene more than 50 years ago. I was giving my grandad a hug and a man walked past smoking a roll up. Whenever, I smell smoke I am reminded of a special moment only grandchildren with special grandparents will understand.

When I smell Dettol I am reminded of the pain of grazing my knee, something that happened a lot when I was a child.

You can see that memories can invoke pain quite easily just as they can bring moments of joy.

Histamine's ability to initiate pain, which is widespread, as well as activate other substances which cause pain, effect inflammation in the brain. Our brain's remarkable ability to store memories more than adequately address how histamine and histamine intolerance can be responsible for symptoms of FMS.

The continuing research into FMS is to be applauded as it can now be seen as a real disease which impacts greatly on the quality of the sufferer's life and that of their family.

The Serine Hypothesis

A number of studies have found low levels of an amino acid, called serine, in people with fibromyalgia syndrome.

 Serine is a non-essential amino acid that is obtained from another amino acid called glycine. It is essential for proper functioning of the brain and is useful in seizure and sleep disorders as it has a calming action.

Serine also makes another well-known amino acid, called tryptophan. Tryptophan is an essential amino acid used to make serotonin which is involved in mood regulation. A lack of tryptophan is believed to cause depression, insomnia and anxiety.

In addition, serine helps to promote muscle mass in the body due to its ability to absorb creatine which helps to build and maintain muscle.

Moreover, it helps to regulate the immune system.

For serine to be produced in the body the co-factors vitamin B complex and folic acid are required. Even then, D-Serine is poorly absorbed when taken orally.

L-Serine has a much better absorption rate. However, supplementation may be useful if a serine deficiency is suspected. The body and its metabolic pathways are complex and not all the steps necessary for serine creation may be completed satisfactorily leading to a serine deficiency.

Dr Rosemary Vallings, a New Zealand GP, recounted her informal study[8] at an Australian conference of six CFIDS patients, who were found to have low urinary levels of serine. After

---

[8] https://www.prohealth.com/library/l-serine-treatment-for-chronic-fatigue-syndrome-cfids-11562

one month five of the six patients reported improvements in:

- Joints and muscles
- Ear, nose and throat
- Energy
- Digestive tract

Dr Vallings supplemented her patients with 500mg of serine, twice daily.

L-serine and D-serine have differing functions as well as overlapping ones. L-serine is converted to the D form by an enzyme.

D-serine is found in the brain and helps information processing. As such a lack of this amino acid can be seen to contribute to the brain fog that so many with FMS complain of.

L-serine assists in increasing levels of creatine. Creatine helps to increase muscle mass in the body.

As some serine will be converted to glycine which is a powerful pain reliever, it has the potential to relieve the pain found in fibromyalgia syndrome *if a serine deficiency is ascertained to be the cause of it.*

Serine can be obtained from all animal foods as well as peanuts and soy products. As [9]retro-conversion with glycine occurs, then sources of glycine such as bone stock, will be a readily available source of a precursor to serine provided vitamin B and folic acid are provided in the diet.

Fibromyalgia and Coenzyme Q10 Deficiency

Coenzyme Q10 is a powerful antioxidant. It is a product of a metabolic pathway known as the Mevalonate Pathway. It helps transport electrons in the mitochondrial respiratory chain.

Mitochondria are tiny powerhouses found in every cell. They are essential for life. Any blockage to their activity results the dysfunction

---

[9] Retroversion is a process whereby substances can convert back to each other as and when the body requires.

of the mitochondria and subsequently, oxidative damage.

We can get some sort of a sense of how coenzyme Q10 impacts us by the effects shown on individuals who are statin users. Statins block the production of coenzyme Q10.   One of the well-known side effects of statins is muscle pain and stiffness which is not unlike the muscular pain and stiffness found in fibromyalgia syndrome.

In a study,[10] five individuals with fibromyalgia syndrome scored their pain on a Visual Analogous Scale of Pain. They were given 300mg of coenzyme Q10 daily for nine months and, after this time, a statistically significant improvement was found.

Similar studies have replicated these results and highlighted that symptoms of tiredness, morning fatigue and pain were statistically significantly reduced.

---

[10] https://www.ncbi.nlm.nih.gov/pubmed/21496502

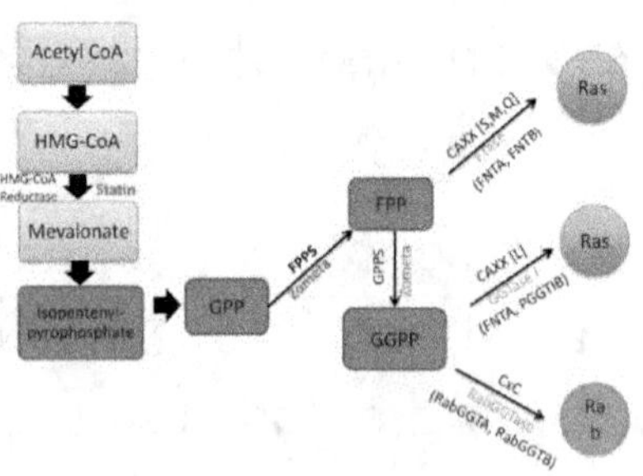

The Mevalonate pathway synthesises coenzyme Q10

Coenzyme Q10 deficiency becomes more marked as we age. This occurs for a number of reasons.

- We eat less as we age so our intake of nutrients is reduced
- We absorb less of the nutrients that we do ingest

In addition, many of the foods containing the highest amounts of this antioxidant are no longer eaten. These foods include organ meats like liver and kidney. As these foods fell out of favour it was noticeable that cases of fibromyalgia syndrome rose.

Other good sources of Q10 are pork, beef and chicken, fatty fish, broccoli and cauliflower and legumes.

Supplementation with coenzyme Q10 should always be considered if an individual has fibromyalgia syndrome, takes statins or is over forty years old. Those who eat little of the foods that contain this antioxidant would be wise to supplement.

Fibromyalgia and hidden   Ehlers Danlos Syndrome

Elhers Danlos Syndrome is the connective tissue disorder that most people have never heard of. There are a number of subtypes but really what concerns us here is that it is a systemic disorder. When things go wrong, then the effects will be felt, to some greater or lesser degree, all over the body.

EDS is characterised by a zebra. The idea behind this is that everyone recognises a zebra but no two zebras have identical stripes. In the same way EDS can manifest itself in many different ways.

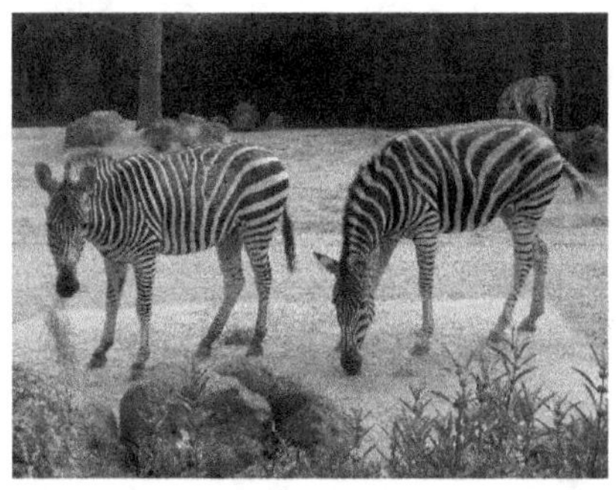

Connective tissue is formed from collagen and is found in skin, bone, cartilage muscles, tendons, ligaments and so on. It forms part of every organ.

Without proper collagen synthesis then any part of the body can suffer. Muscle aches and pains are not uncommon. Digestive issues occur due to the laxity of tissue in the bowel leading to gastroparesis and chronic constipation.

Fatigue is a debilitating symptom. The appearance of Raynaud's is significantly increased. Headaches manifest themselves on a daily basis.

Sadly, it takes on average nineteen years for someone to be diagnosed with Ehlers Danlos Syndrome. The very diversity and apparently unrelated symptoms often lead to doctors scratching their heads wondering what is going on.

When a physical cause cannot be found for the pain the patient is complaining of, then the doctor generally reverts back to that good old favourite of a mental illness at play.

While anxiety and depression may well result of constant pain and discomfort it is not the initiating cause.

I have often said that I would like to see posters up in doctors' surgeries waiting rooms showing some of the unusual signs of EDS.

One of these is the ability to touch your thumb on the wrist of the same side. Most people will know if they can do this –it was probably one of their party pieces when they were younger but they will not know that it is likely that it is a sign of   EDS

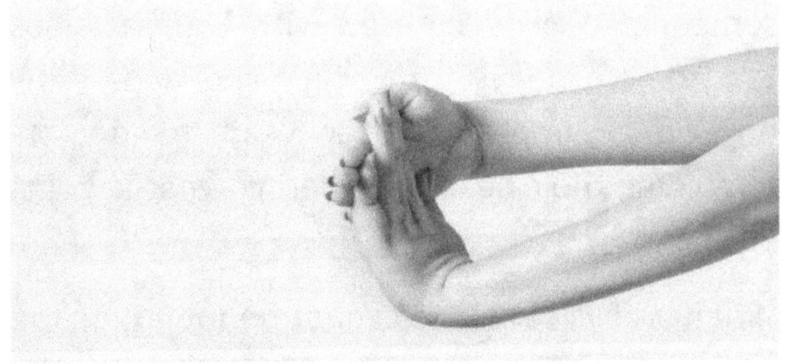

Lax joints are a hallmark of Ehlers Danlos Syndrome.

It is always worth looking on the EDS website - which gives the diagnostic criteria for EDS – to see if some of the criteria apply to you. If they do, then make an appointment with your GP who will likely refer you to a rheumatologist.

The Dangers of Manufactured Citric Acid (MCA)

As always, there can be more than one cause of any manifestation of a condition. During my research I happened to have my attention drawn to Manufactured Citric Acid and spent weeks following this through as it seemed to have implications for many chronic diseases such asthma, lymphoedema, lipoedema, Alzheimer's disease, arthritis, allergies and gastrointestinal disturbance. This is not a definitive list. Indeed, my attention was first turned towards the problems with MCA when I was advising someone on the benefits of real – not manufactured citric acid – in aiding gut motility.

The discovery of citric acid was credited to an alchemist Jabir ibn Hayaan going as far back at the 8th century. However, it was not isolated in its pure form until nine centuries later when Carl Steele crystallised it from lemon juice in 1784.

The lemon juice was imported from Italy and peak production occurred in 1915-1916 after which it began to decline due to cost.

The change from the crystallisation of citric to a fermentation process occurred in 1919 in Belgium using the mould known as penicillium. However, the duration of fermentation and the risk of contamination meant that the use of penicillium was abandoned.

In 1917, James Currie – an American food chemist – discovered that the mould *Aspergillus niger* could produce cost effective amounts of citric acid using molasses as the raw material.

In 1919, Pfizer adopted this method and began to produce citric acid using *Aspergillus niger*. This method is used today and we refer to this citric acid as manufactured citric acid or MCA.

The Food Standards Agency normally evaluates food additives for safety and they are given GRAS status – Generally Recognised as Safe. However, the Food Additives Amendment 1958 excluded any additives – including MCA – that were in use before 1958 that had not appeared to have demonstrated harm.

This does not mean that it does not cause harm. Some conditions take many years to diagnose and even so, the underlying cause may still be unknown.

99% of citric acid used today is the MCA sort. It is an ubiquitous substance and arguably the most common food additive. It is used to stabilise and preserve the active ingredients.

The global market growth and the related use of citric acid is undoubtedly driven by concomitant growth in pharmaceuticals, cosmetics and processed foods.

It can be found in:

Processed and prepared foods

Carbonated beverages, fruit and energy drinks

Nutritional supplements and vitamins

Common snacks

Confectionary

Pharmaceuticals

Canned fruit and veg

It is also used in non-food stuffs as it is a useful disinfectant against many viruses and bacteria.

Currently, the market share of MCA appears to be taken by:

Food and beverages	70%
Pharmaceuticals and cosmetics	20%
Cleaning and softening agents	10%

In a research paper[11] the potential harms of MCA are raised. The authors cite four case reports of individuals who demonstrate symptoms which include:

Joint pain with swelling and stiffness, muscular pain, dyspnea, abdominal cramping, and

---

[11] https://www.ncbi.nlm.nih.gov/pmc/articles/PMC6097542/

enervation that started within 2-12 hours of ingesting anything which contained MCA.

The severity of symptoms appears to be the deciding factor in how long before they resolve which could be anywhere from 8-72 hours.

The case participants did not know beforehand which foods contained MCA yet were able to correctly identify, based on symptoms, those which were.

It was found that the ingestion of natural forms of citric acid did not result in such symptoms.

Aspergillus niger is thermos tolerant and cannot be killed. Even when it is the end products is still pro-inflammatory. It is extremely likely that there are contaminants from production.

China is the largest producer of MCA and continues to expand as demand expects. Auto immune disorders and allergies have been found to be increasing in parallel.

Indeed, some of other conditions that appear to be related to MCA ingestion are:

ASD, juvenile idiopathic arthritis, fibromyalgia as well as allergies and angieoedema type conditions and neurological conditions.

Late onset Alzheimer's disease is associated with reduced nicotinamide adenosine triphosphate (NAD) metabolism and an altered citric acid cycle also known as the TCA or the tricarboxylic acid cycle.

As it is MCA that is found in pharmaceutical drugs, then the impact of taking such drugs cannot be ignored.

Serious side effects are outlined[12] and include the citric acid which forms part of potassium citrate and sodium citrate too. This include numbness, tingly feeling, swelling or rapid weight gain, muscle twitching, cramps, fast or slow heartbeat, confusion, mood changes, bloody or tarry stools, severe stomach pain, ongoing diarrhoea or seizures.

---

[12] https://www.uofmhealth.org/health-library/d03951a1

The bone and muscle juddering pain of Vitamin D deficiency

Anyone who has read any of my other books will know that I am passionate about educating people about the perils of vitamin D deficiency.

What most people don't know is that a shortage of vitamin D can result in deep and gnawing bone pain which is not resolved when analgesics are taken. It is also the cause of fatigue and headaches, constipation, anxiety and depression.

In fact, the very symptoms that trouble people with FMS.

Approximately 80% of the world population are deficient in this vitamin which is required for strong bones as well as regulating inflammation.

It is one of the most difficult of vitamins to take in sufficient quantities through the diet. Foods containing vitamin D are limited and what foods there are do not contain great amounts.

As we get older we are less likely to absorb the nutrients from our diet. Vitamin D is no different so increasing age is a risk factor for a deficiency of vitamin D.

Most of our vitamin D is taken in through the action of the sun's rays on the skin but even this process becomes less efficient as we age.

Supplementation of 2000 IU's is recommended daily unless you have been out in the summer sun and had adequate exposure to the sun's rays and then you do not need to take it.

In the winter between the end of September and the beginning of April, 5000 IU's is beneficial.

This should be taken in its active form D3 rather than the inactive form, D2. The latter requires a number of steps to be converted to the active form. As age progresses, the conversion process is likely to be less effective.

Dietary sources of vitamin D are irradiated mushrooms, eggs and oily fish. However, supplementation of vitamin D should only be taken in conjunction with adequate vitamin K2. Vitamin K2 is found in fermented foods including hard cheese and kefir.

My final thoughts on the subject of FMS and CFS rest on whether we should be looking for one underlying cause or whether the symptoms manifested in a number of individuals are the result of a   number of different conditions.

The body is, after all, a wonderfully complex piece of machinery directed by thousands of genes which are influenced by the ever changing environment.

Diseases come and go depending on environmental conditions but many vastly different conditions produce similar symptoms.

Research has always looked into causes that are easy to study. Money is a factor in deciding what the areas of investigation into a condition should be.

 However, the reality is that the answer to our pain and fatigue may be one of extreme complexity and, as such, may never attract funding for further investigation.

This is frustrating when people want answers and a quick fix prescription as that may not be forthcoming but it does not stop us from listening to our bodies closely,

I know that if I eat dark chocolate, I will have a migraine. If I eat tomatoes, my elbow will start itching (yes, really!)

Many of us successfully self-diagnose. We identify patterns and begin to make connections and adjustments to relieve symptoms. This is one of the most useful tools that you can use and it works.

So, in the absence of the likely known causes of the syndrome as mentioned in earlier parts of this book, being responsible for FMS, keep a diary and jot down activities and diet to try and establish a connection.

Always rate your stress levels. Every single person that I know with FMS has stressful events going on in their life that would floor most people.

Often they don't recognise this because the stressful event has become woven into their lives and they have forgotten what life was like before then.

My hope is that you will uncover the reason behind the symptoms that you have so that you can participate fully into life with joy and vigour.

Thank you for purchasing this book. Every time a book is purchased, a donation is made to one of the charities I am currently supporting. These can be found on my author's website. See below.

Other Health Related Books by the Author

- **The Reluctant Bowel**
- **A Weighty Issue**
- **Sleep, Perchance to Dream**
- **The Journey: EDS and chronic pain**

- **The MND diet: using nutrition to slow down the progress of neurodegeneration**
- **A Necessary Sorrow**
- **Taking another Road: Pain: its causes and what can be done about it.**
- **Osteoarthritis**
- **Treat infection naturally**
- **Treatment strategy for Migraine**
- **The Metabolic Syndrome Diet**
- **EDS and Weight Gain**
- **Journey through pneumonia**
- **Beat hypertension easily using nutrition**

These can be found here on the author's page

https://www.amazon.co.uk/-/e/B07BPQZ5CD

You may also be interested in the semi-autobiographical trilogy of the authors life found in these three books

- The Prejudged
- Where the Blackbird Never Sings

- A Summer's Symphony

And the author's children's books

- Fanny and Victorian Jack
- Fanny and the Gamekeeper's Cottage